MY DOWNWARD

SPIRAL

TO FREEDOM

BY MARIA ROBERTS

My Downward Spiral to Freedom

© 2020 by Maria Roberts

Published in Hampton, VA, by Fruition Publishing Concierge Services. Fruition Publishing Concierge Services is a division of Alesha Brown, LLC.

Fruition Publishing Concierge Services can bring authors to your live event. For more information or to book an event, visit Fruition Publishing Concierge Services at:

www.FruitionPublishing.com

ISBN: 978-1-954486-00-3 Paperback

ISBN: 978-1-954486-01-0 eBook

Library of Congress Control Number: 2020925938

Unless otherwise noted, all scriptures are from The Holy Bible, New International Version. (1984). Grand Rapids: Zondervan Publishing House.

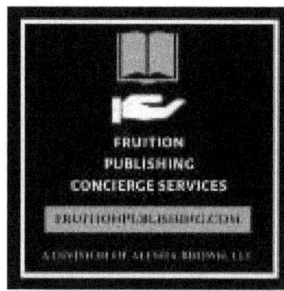

FRUITION
PUBLISHING
CONCIERGE SERVICES

FRUITIONPUBLISHING.COM

A DIVISION OF ALESHA BROWN, LLC

DEDICATION

**To those who suffer hopelessly from the disease of
addiction, may you find hope and freedom.**

TABLE OF CONTENTS

INTRODUCTION

It's easy to talk about the wonderful things that happen on this journey called life, but the true tests come when you reveal the darkest part of your story. The part you wish you could just leave out or skip over. The part that may cause people to look at you differently. The part that you would rather forget, but ultimately there is no forgetting the part that makes you who you are. We are our story—the light and the dark.

The darkest part of my story involves making a choice that would send me spiraling into the grips of drug addiction. Addiction took me on a roller coaster ride that went from intriguing to my worst nightmare. In an instant, my life was on a downward spiral that I thought would lead to my death. Addiction changed my life forever!

THE BEGINNING

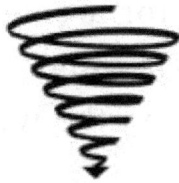

I remember the first time I smoked crack cocaine–it was in the late 1980s. I was driving from New York to Virginia and I hit a laced joint. The weed had been sprinkled with crushed crack cocaine and I absolutely loved it. I was an occasional weed smoker at the time, but this was something totally different and I had to have more.

I remember stopping to get more before I continued my trip to Virginia. I was going to Virginia to see my children. I had moved to New York to pursue modeling and my children were still in Virginia. I remember always being excited about coming home to see them, but the moment I hit that laced joint, that all changed.

My mind went automatically to the drug. I could not travel without it. I had absolutely no idea what that one moment would cost me.

I did some on-call modeling during the day with an agency in New York City and I had a pretty good job working the 3rd shift for a company in Upstate New York. Financially I was good. I worked hard during the week and got high on the weekends.

Within six months, I started getting high during the week before working 3rd shift and I went to very few model calls during the day. My modeling dream was deferred. I continued working the 3rd shift job, most of the time high because that's the only way I could have money to get more. It was my means to an end! My life was a whirlwind of working and getting high.

I didn't even commute to Virginia on a regular basis to see my kids anymore; I was too busy. However, when I did, I would make sure I had plenty of drugs to travel with. I simply loved being high and I had no idea that I was addicted. I thought I was just "partying."

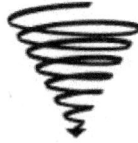

The New York "party" ended in less than two years when I totaled my car and moved back to Virginia. Back in Virginia, things were much slower but my craving to get high hadn't changed. What did change is that I couldn't smoke in front of my kids and I didn't have the 3rd shift job nor the freedom that I had in New York. I had to work a 1st shift job while being a full-time mother, which really put a damper on my partying schedule. I found myself sneaking to smoke in the bathroom at home and even in the car at work.

The "party" wasn't fun anymore and the straw that broke the camel's back was when I started missing events in my children's life—dipping out on birthday parties and not being present for Mother's Day. For the first time, I realized that I was in trouble and I needed help. I decided to check into an inpatient rehabilitation hospital. I managed to stay clean for five years until my father passed away.

My father's passing was a pain that I could not handle sober. I immediately wanted to get high and that is exactly what I did. That time, my addiction took me from having a job and a family to being a homeless prostitute in a matter of five years. My addiction was all I had. I lived to get high and soon came to believe that I would die getting high.

The next few chapters will unveil to you a day in the life of a crack-addicted prostitute. My life, the part that most people would never reveal, and the dark side of my life journey to the road to true freedom.

FEEDING MY ADDICTION

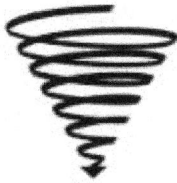

It would be sunrise in a couple of hours and I hadn't been to sleep. I had spent the last hour tripping while watching the roaches run back and forth on the ceiling. More days than not started out this way.

Night after night, the night would turn to morning and I would never experience sleep. I was always happy when 5 am would come around because I would have a better chance to make some money so I could get my fix. Even though it was cold outside, I had to go get more crack if I wanted to stay inside where it was warm and to take care of my nagging addiction.

The houseman, the owner of the house where I was at, was an addict too and no one could stay in his house for free. He required payment which was either crack or cash-no *shorts*. I hadn't given him anything in nearly three hours, but luckily he had fallen asleep.

I knew that I needed to hit the street soon because the workers would start driving and I could stop one of them if I hurried. Someone would surely be looking for me to make them happy before they went to work and, most assuredly, I would be looking for them to make me happy before they went to work. I had what they wanted and they had what I wanted so the stroll would begin.

I pulled out my baby wipes and went to the bathroom to try to freshen up a little bit. There was no running water in the house so that was my only resource. I detangled my wig with my fingers, wiped my face off, and put on a little face powder. I looked through my backpack to see if I had anything clean enough to change into or if I needed to keep on what I had. After a brief look inside, I decided to keep what I had on. I grabbed my coat and I was ready for the day. Little did I know that would be my last day out.

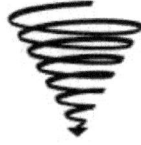

It was a cold winter morning, but my adrenaline was so high that I did not feel the cold. I was excited! I was on a mission, a money mission.

It was time to hit the block. Time for work—turning tricks to support my addiction. I had been on the stroll for more than five hours. The stroll was what we called the street we walked up and down to get work. The worst part of the stroll for me was it was the main street in the neighborhood that I grew up. I hated the fact that people knew me from before. They knew my parents and surely wondered how I ended up like that. What people thought really didn't matter, but I hated that my mom lived in the neighborhood.

I walked the stroll to support my crack addiction, but it wasn't always that way. Initially, I dated a drug dealer and I worked a regular job. Crack was so easily available that I didn't even know I was addicted until he got locked up. That's when reality set in. I was an addict and I would do anything to feed my addiction.

When I got outside, the sun hadn't come up yet. It was prime time to start walking down to where I knew one of my regulars would be looking for me before he went to work.

As I approached the block I saw his white truck going by. I wasn't sure if he saw me so I ran to the block really quick and began to walk in the direction that he was traveling. Then I saw his brake lights come on and then his signal light. I was in business!

He was one of my regulars and I knew once we were done with business, I would walk away with enough cash to score enough to last me a few hours. Plus, if he was in a good mood he would also give me a tip, but the best part of dealing with Mr. White Truck was he always let me score first so I could take a hit before my work began.

Mr. White Truck was Caucasian, in his early 30, and I had been knowing him for three years. When I think about it, most of my customers were white. He was a blue-collar worker, most of the time looking pretty dirty in his blue uniform. His potbelly hung down over his pants, but he was always kind to me, never blatantly demeaning.

I had robbed him a few months back when we went to a hotel. He wanted me to spend the whole night, but I had grown to hate being in hotels for extended periods of time. I would get so paranoid. I always felt like someone was watching or they could smell in the hallway when I took a hit. I couldn't enjoy my high, constantly looking out of the peephole.

Plus, he had the audacity to take a shower and leave his wallet right on the dresser. Who does that? Needless to say, I robbed him and ran. He had like $500 in his wallet. I left him $200 because he really was a nice guy.

I remember the first time I saw him after that. I ran as fast as I could, but he followed me and pulled into a street right in front of me. So I went ahead and confronted him. Surprisingly he just asked me why I did that to him and I looked him straight in his eyes and said, "I'm an addict. What did you think would happen?" He laughed and said, "What are you doing now?" We continued with business as usual.

Lucky for me, today was no different. He gave me a hundred-dollar bill and we went down the block where all the drug dealers hung out. I was able to score enough to be set for a few hours.

After scoring, I quickly pulled out my stem and loaded it for my first hit of the day as he drove to our normal spot in the back of the graveyard. I remember the first time we went to the graveyard; it was five or six years prior to that day. When he turned into the graveyard, I was like "No, no, no, no, no. We can't go in there because my dad is buried out there."

It's crazy to think about it because as the years went by and my addiction progressed, I didn't care where we went as long as I got the money and my drugs. After our business, I had Mr. White Truck drop me off at the same house I had left from that morning.

SMOKE SOME, SELL SOME

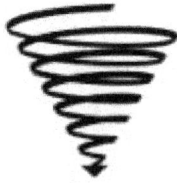

The houseman was on the porch when I got back. I told him to come on inside because we had a nice score. I broke him off; that would allow me to stay at least 2 1/2 hours. I had a good amount left for myself, but with my habit, I would back on the stroll sooner than later. That's the nature of the beast!

I went into the first bedroom of the houseman's home and broke my score up into pieces. It was my intention to sell some and smoke. I always tried to do that because at least I'd have money left over to score again and perhaps I wouldn't have to go back on the stroll as often. Well, that was my rationale.

I loved having time alone to smoke in the morning, especially after waiting so long during the night to be able to get some work and score again. I tried to savor every hit and lay back and relax. Most of the time when I got high I wasn't a paranoid smoker. Unlike some crack smokers, I didn't feel the need to constantly look out the window or I think someone was coming to get me or something bad was about to happen.

I actually enjoyed getting high—it was my escape from reality. The reality that I had lost everything and ruined my life to become a drug addict. Never in a million years did I picture my life ending up like this.

Nevertheless, the house that I was at was really comfortable for me that morning because I had paid the houseman well so I knew that he would not allow anyone to disturb me. Actually, he was too busy getting high himself and reaping the benefits of other people that were coming through to get high. Everyone that came in had to break him off first before they could settle down. I often wished that I had my own house so I could just sit there and get high off of everybody else's work, but that's not my story. I had to work hard for every hit I took.

During the time that I was in the room, I sold enough to make $80. I had originally broken enough pieces to make $100, but $80 was better than nothing and I was actually surprised that I didn't smoke all of the ones that I intended to sell. I was ahead of the game!

I needed to go back out on the block real quick to get at least $20 to add to the $80 I made so I could score a nice piece again. That was the plan! So, I went once again to the bathroom, took out some baby wipes to freshen up. (The water had actually been turned off for a couple of months.) After a quick clean up, back on the stroll I went.

EASY MONEY

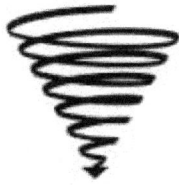

It was still pretty cold out. I walked for about 15 minutes before I got some work.

This time it was Benz that I didn't recognize but it passed me and turned on the next block up and stopped. I knew that was my signal, so I ran over and quickly jumped in.

To my surprise, it was an older gentleman. I asked him what was his pleasure. He surprisingly told me that he just wanted my company while he took care of himself. Now that was a pretty weird request, but nonetheless, I was elated because it would cost him $100 and I didn't have to do anything.

He was an older man that I hadn't seen on the block before and he could have very well been the police, but my instincts told me that he was just a quick way to make some quick money. I'm guessing he was in his late 50s; he had on a dress shirt and tie and khaki pants.

He looked like a businessman, so I knew that he definitely could afford $100. He agreed and paid me—I always got paid upfront.

I told him to drive down the street and just park between two parked cars. I knew this wouldn't take long. He parked and in less than three minutes, I exited his car. I didn't know him so I didn't trust him to drop me off anywhere, so I just got out of his car, grateful for the easy money. Now I had $180 and my greedy thinking was that if I could just stay on the stroll a little longer, I would be able to score a really nice piece.

I was still feeling pretty good after my morning smoke session that I had had earlier, so I didn't really feel the urge to take a hit right away. As long as it didn't take too long, I would be okay. I have been on the street long enough to know how to work smart and score big. Granted it didn't always turn out that way. Some days all I could get was $20 work and score $20 pieces all day long. At the end of the day, I would be exhausted but today had been a good day so far.

I walked up the block towards the corner where the dope boy was that I scored from earlier, hoping I'd catch a quick trick on the way. On my way, I stopped at this guy's house that was on disability. He was a cheap trick, but I would go to him when I was in a bind or if I needed a little quick money. Since the next day was the 1st of the month and sometimes he got his check early, I decided to try my luck.

I rang the doorbell and I was in business. He was straight; he had gotten his check a day early!

As usual, he tried to convince me to take care of him for $20. No way José. I wasn't in that much of a bind but I was in a hurry. My high was gone now and I needed a hit!

Needless to say, I got $40 from him and finished him off fast. I liked coming to his house because I could use his phone to call the dope man. I made my call and told the dope boy to meet me back at the house where I was renting the room that morning.

I was about four blocks from the house where I started my day, so I walked back almost running. I needed a hit! When I got back to the house, I told the houseman that the dope boy was on his way, then I went into the bedroom and pushed my stem to get a hit from the crack residue that had built up on the sides of the glass earlier. I was able to get a pretty good hit from the residue, enough to keep me calm while I waited. It seemed like I waited an eternity, but it actually had only been 15 minutes before the dope man showed up.

I bought a nice piece with $200, but unfortunately for me, the dope man was a regular customer as well. After I scored, he pulled out a condom, walked over to the houseman, and broke him off to use the room for a minute. Then he walked towards the bedroom and motioned me to join him.

Granted this would earn me more crack, but I needed a real hit bad and I already had crack so I didn't need him! I told him I'd get with him later, but he never ever took 'no' for an answer. I pushed my luck a little further and asked him if I could go in the bathroom for a second, that way I could sneak a hit first. Of course, he didn't agree with that either.

I had watched the dope game change immensely over the years. It went from scoring from older drug dealers that had fine houses and luxury cars to scoring from these young street corner thugs who thought they ran the world. Needless to say, he pulled me into the room, slammed the door, and threw me on the bed. He went in his pocket and broke me off. After about five minutes we were all done and he exited the bedroom.

I could finally take a hit. I was loading my stem when the houseman busted in the room. "Did you forget something?" I broke him off another gram and looked up to see that he still had his hand out. He wanted me to pay him for using the room for work even though the dope boy had just paid him earlier.

At this point, all I knew was that I needed a hit bad, so I gave him the crumbs from the bottom of the bag. He smiled and took his exit.

Finally, I could get high in peace! It had been quite a successful day. I had a really nice score so I decided to try and take my time. After a satisfying hit, I broke up some pieces to sell, leaving me a good amount to smoke. I was literally on cloud nine.

I got my mirror and razor blade out and set myself up for a personal party. I loaded my stem, put the lighter to it, and watched the smoke fill the room over and over again. I was having a ball! Nobody was knocking on the door. It was perfect while it lasted.

LET'S PARTY

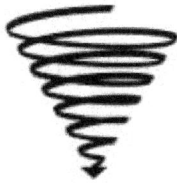

I did well smoking by myself for an hour or so, but unfortunately, I hated to smoke longer than that by myself. It was like I got lonely or something, so I invited the houseman into the room to smoke with me. Between the two of us, we had enough for a serious afternoon party, so we decided to make it a *Do Not Disturb* party.

He got his boy, the guy that cooks and cleans for him, to watch the front door. We agreed that we would only answer the door for a sale $20 or higher and we would rotate the sales to make it fair.

The party was on. We both took our clothes off because he liked to get naked while we got high and

I didn't mind because nothing really happened—we just got high naked.

The houseman and I had known each other for a long time. Actually, he was one of the first people I met when I started getting high in Virginia so we had known each other for years. Although he was an addict himself, we had a special bond. He knew I wasn't a moocher or a beggar. If I was in the house, I was pulling my own weight.

The relationship that the houseman and I had formed made it easier for me when I was in a bind, unable to pay him to stay inside. He rarely would turn me away from staying in even when I didn't have crack or cash. However, I had learned early in the game not to take his kindness for weakness.

I knew him before his crack addiction and he was a totally different person. He was a successful businessman with a beautiful home and nice cars. It's unbelievable how crack can transform a person!

Shoot, look at me. I was married with three kids, college-educated, and living in a nice home with a good job and car. This was all BC: Before Crack! Now

I was homeless and on the street tricking to support my addiction. Who knew?

During our private party, we had several knocks on the door for sales. I actually sold all that I broke off earlier. So I asked the houseman to make a call so I could get more to continue our party! He had also sold a good amount so we decided to put our money together.

We scored enough to keep me inside at least until sunset, but things didn't work out that way. Our private party was going good for a while until the houseman's interests in getting high with me alone started to dwindle.

Someone knocked on the door and it was a young lady that he fancied. She wanted to score a $20 piece. Instead of breaking her off at the door, he invited her in. That young lady was someone that I had known for a very long time as well. She actually taught me everything that I knew about working the street. Nonetheless, we both had the same mission to get high for as long as possible with minimal work and minimal distraction. It was not possible for both of us to be successful in the same room, especially when I was holding a good amount and all she had to offer was a $20 piece.

Now things were getting messy. Our twosome was now a threesome! She got undressed and proceeded to smoke her piece, then she revealed that she had another $100. I knew it wasn't like her to just have $20, but I thought we all have bad days sometimes, but she was always a slick one!

She was one of the houseman's favorite girls and she tried to convince him to let her score from him instead of calling the dope boys. It wasn't advantageous for a smoker to sell weight because it left you with less money and less product.

He actually didn't have enough left to sell her, so he looked at me. Listen, there was no way I was going to sell her a $100 piece when I could get $300 selling it broken up or just smoke it myself! Duh!

Eventually, the houseman called the dope boy to come back for her and she scored from him. After she scored she made herself right at home, sitting on the bed with both of us. I was never much for a threesome, especially when I had my own supply. That's quite different than if I didn't have anything and I was joining a party to get high, so of course, I wasn't very happy with this new arrangement.

I wasn't stupid though. That time, when I prepared the mirror, I only broke off three small hits and stuffed the rest deep in my shoe. In turn, the young lady that had joined us and the houseman did the same. They both broke off three small hits as well. I picked up a hit and slid my feet into my shoes. I proceeded to get up from the bed and go over to the chair that was located near the door and took my hit.

The houseman and his new company were quite involved with one another and he didn't even look up when there were knocks at the door for sales. I was able to make $80 in sales from what I had in my shoe. It was time to make my exit.

A CHANGE OF SCENERY

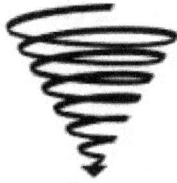

By the time they ran out, I had managed to make $120 without the houseman knowing and enough left to offer them both a hit. Then I kindly got dressed and told the houseman that I had a date, but I'd be back.

I handed him a hit while I wrapped up my stem and stuffed it in my bra. Then I made a quick exit out of the room and out the front door before the houseman could get dressed and come after me. When I gave him the hit, I'm sure he was wondering if I still had dope left or money.

Now I was outside high with drugs on me. That was not a good look and I didn't really have a date. I needed to think of someplace to go fast. I didn't want to be on the street too long with drugs and paraphernalia on me.

The closest crack house to sit and smoke was like six blocks away. I started a brisk walk in that direction. It was just getting dark outside so that made me feel really paranoid because the cops patrolled more heavily at night. I didn't hit the main strip while I was walking. I took the side streets and came up on the crack house from the back roads.

This particular crack house was initially a very tough place for me to go to because it was actually the home of one of my best childhood friends. I remember the first time that I was escorted over there to get high. When we pulled up in front of the house, I couldn't believe that this was where we were going. I had spent numerous days during my elementary school years through my high school years visiting my friend and her parents at this house. The memories were overwhelming. But just like the cemetery, the more my addiction progressed, my "dis-ease" soon subsided because I needed somewhere to score and somewhere to get high.

I was in luck: the house lady answered the door right away when I knocked and I quickly stepped in. She was smiling ear to ear because she knew whenever she saw me I came bearing gifts. I told her, "Let's slip into the backroom real quick." (The front end of the house was filled with people laying on the sofa, sitting at the kitchen table, and just standing around.)

I didn't smell much crack smoke so I knew that more than likely no one had anything and I would be bombarded with beggars if I didn't move fast. She grabbed my hand and we went straight to the backroom. I noticed that one of the dope boys was in her living room so I told her to have him come to the backroom because I wanted to score.

Automatically, straight off the bat, he thought that I wanted to work. He broke her off, pushed her out the door, and closed the door behind her. Then he broke me off and took his condom out. It was a different dope boy from earlier, but the same game. So here we go again!

I didn't argue. I knew it wouldn't take long to finish him off because he was nervous being confined in her backroom for a long period of time. This house was nothing like that other house that I had been at. It definitely wasn't safe for him to be in the backroom for a long period of time. After business was done, I told him I wanted to score dime weight. Unfortunately, he didn't sell weight.

Now I was in a bind because he asked me if I wanted to score some $20 pieces and he'd throw in an extra one, but I had the pieces he had just paid me with plus so I wasn't pressed to spend my money frivolously. I was straight! I was having too good of a day to start scoring small weight, so I just scored one $20 piece from him so he could get out of my face. I knew I had to score something or he would be mad.

After I scored the $20 piece, I quickly made my exit out of the room before he could try to take the money from me and force me to get all $20s. I made a beeline straight for the front door. The house lady came running out after me. Just when I was getting ready to tell her I'd be back, a car pulled up and the dope boy came out of the house and got in the car. They pulled off, so I felt safe to go back inside.

Back inside, I told her that she would have to clear some of those people out of the house if she wanted me to stay. Of course, she wanted me to stay because my reputation was one of always having crack or money. I wasn't one that many people turned away. She proceeded to clear the house and put both locks on the front door and secure the back door. My girl! I used her phone to call my boy that I knew sold weight; he was right down the street so he was there within three minutes. Now I had a nice amount and I was back in business, ready to chill. That day continued to be a good day.

After she escorted the dope boy out, we went to the back bedroom where I broke her off and told her to give me an hour without being disturbed. She kindly obliged and I took off my coat, pulled my stem out of my bra, and quieted my nerves with a nice big hit. One thing I knew about this house lady was that she got very paranoid when she got high and she liked to drink. It wouldn't be long before she let somebody in the house and they would disturb my peace, so I didn't get too comfortable. I knew without a doubt that even though I had paid her to give me an hour, she would be back before the hour was up.

After I enjoyed a couple of good hits, I pulled my baby wipes out of my backpack so I could start freshening up to hit the block before she came back in. Sure enough, in less than 45 minutes, she was back knocking on the door asking me did I have a hit for her! I went ahead and gave her another hit, just enough to give me time to get ready to leave. I wrapped the rest up in a tissue and put it in my underwear. I pushed the chore boy from one end of my stem to the other to get a hit off of all the crack residue that had built up. It was one of the most amazing pushes that I had ever hit. Unfortunately, I froze and couldn't move.

In my mind, I knew that I needed to put my coat on so that I could leave, but I was tripping too hard. I couldn't leave yet and I was too paranoid to stay in the backroom, so I went out front still holding my stem in a daze. One of my glaring thoughts was that I wanted to make sure that I scored from that same guy the rest of the day because he had really good stuff!

When I got to the front room, a young lady came in that wanted to score a $20 piece. I went into the bathroom and took my stash out of my underwear and broke her off. We made the exchange, she broke off the house lady, and then we both went into the backroom together.

I felt better having someone back there with me, plus this young lady had always been kind to me over the years. She always shared a hit with me when I didn't have anything; that was rare. So I would always do the same for her and that's how we built a special bond. I never felt uncomfortable getting high with her; she wasn't a beggar. She worked for hers just like I did and I respected that.

The house lady was still drinking that whole time and her drinking and smoking crack didn't mix. By the time I took another hit and before my friend could finish hers, I heard the house lady yelling and screaming in the front room, "Everybody Out! Everybody Out!" Geez!

My friend and I immediately left out of the backroom. She was like me— avoid confrontation at all costs. Before I could make it to the front door, the house lady was in my face asking me if I had anything left. I shoved my warm stem into my coat pocket and pushed past her out the front door.

Now I was outside again, high with a warm stem in my pocket and drugs on me. Where could I go? I needed to think fast; this was a known crack house and I certainly didn't want the cops to cruise by and see me standing there.

MOTEL HELL

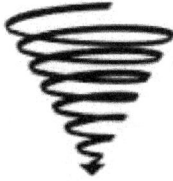

Before I could go into a total panic, one of the guys that had been inside the house getting high came out and he was driving. He asked me if I wanted to ride with him. He said he was going to the ATM and to find someone to score from. I had dealt with him a couple of times. He was pretty new to the scene. I felt sorry for him because he had a good job and he still had a car, but I knew how quickly that could all change.

I climbed into the passenger side of his car and off to the ATM we went. He withdrew $240. I was set again.

While we were driving back from the ATM, I asked him if he wanted a hit. I loaded my stem for him and held the lighter as he took a nice long drag while he was driving. I only felt safe doing that with him because I knew from experience that he didn't trip real hard or get super paranoid when he got high, he just got quiet. I leaned my seat back and took a nice hit as well. He was careful to use his hand to cover the flame so that no one passing by would notice.

When I set back up, I saw that we were heading to the sleaziest hotel near the block. It was actually a motel. I knew I wouldn't be able to stay there long because I was definitely more paranoid whenever I went there just because it was a known crack motel. It's only saving grace was that the rooms were really cheap and, because it was a motel, I didn't have my paranoia of smoke in the hallway like in hotels.

He went into the lobby and secured a room for $40, then parked the car and we went into the room. As always, the room reeked of cigarette smoke. Unlike most of my friends, I didn't smoke cigarettes and I hated the smell. Nevertheless, it was party time and I wanted to get high!

One really good thing about Mr. Good Job and Nice Car was he never wanted to get freaky. We just got high and I made sure he was comfortable. I would always load his stem for him and hold the fire while he took the hit, catering to his every need. I made sure he had some water to drink and I continuously asked him was he okay. He was a nice guy and I just felt sorry for him because I knew where this journey would take him.

I remember when I first started out: I had a good job and a nice car too. However, that didn't last long and, before I knew it, I had quit my job and lost my car. I knew it wouldn't be long before he would be in the same situation and it was ten times worse for men versus women. Men couldn't trick like women to get high. They often ended up getting fired from their jobs, renting their car out to the dope boys until they wrecked it, robbing people and places, selling all their stuff, and writing bad checks. They did anything to get high and, in that regard, they were no different.

Our party only lasted an hour or so. We ran out of drugs and he ran out of money. Not a good combination at all!

He had to get home and get ready for work but he asked me could I get him a front. (He wanted me to see if one of the dope boys would tick him some product until he got paid. It was called a tick because as soon as the dope boy gave you the product, you were on the clock to pay him back.)

Now listen, I loved to get a good tick for myself until I could go make some money but I seldom, if ever, got a tick for somebody else. I had to be real blunt with him—it was time for him to go back to the ATM or go home.

My addiction was serious and I had no time for games. He decided to take the latter option and go home. I wrapped my stem in some toilet tissue and placed it in my bra. Coats on, ready; let's go.

BACK TO THE STROLL

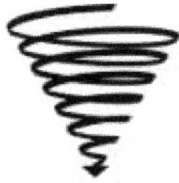

I was out of drugs and I only had $20. It was definitely "time to make the donuts!" I had to think fast so I could get him to drop me off where I would be most successful.

With the next day being the first of the month, I knew my fellow addicts that got a check: Disability, SSI, Retirement, or Other would be getting a 'tick'/credit from the dope man. So I decided to start with them. I figured even if I didn't make any money I could at least party with them and get high for free.

First stop, old man Bird's house. Three addicts lived there and they ALL got a check; they were retired military. They only lived two blocks up the street from where he dropped me off.

First, I gently tapped on the window to Bird's bedroom. "Hey, baby; it's me," I announced. Then I went around to the side door and knocked.

Bird opened the door. He hastily ushered me in. I stepped in and, BINGO, I smelled the illustrious smell of crack in the air! I followed houseman Bird to his room first. He had a small amount of crack on his mirror. I took my coat off, loaded my stem, and took a hit. Judging from how much he had on the mirror, I knew that this wouldn't last long, So I asked Bird to call somebody so I could score with my last $20.

While he was making the call, I went into his roommate's room, but he had a young lady in there so I was too late for that party. I ventured across the hall to the third roommate's room. He was alone and he had a little left so I sat down and took a hit with him. The problem with him was he would get mad paranoid when he got high. I hated getting high with people that were paranoid. Whenever I would make the slightest move, he would ask me what was I doing. Luckily for me, the dope boy got there and I was able to score.

Bird got a small tick from him as well, but, unfortunately, less than an hour later we were out again. I took a chance and I went to both of the other roommate's rooms but they were out as well. This was bad news!

I really thought that the party would have lasted a lot longer because it was three of them in the house, but they had been getting ticks all day. They all started asking me if I knew where they could get another tick from until tomorrow. I did try to call a few people but no one was willing to come out for a tick.

Needless to say, what had been a good day for me was looking pretty bleak. I must admit that at that point it had been a very long day. I had smoked a lot and probably could've passed out at Bird's house until daybreak. The problem was that I didn't want to sleep there because it smelled like urine. When I was high I didn't notice the odor quite so much, but the minute I started coming down, it was unbearable. I had to get out of there. I had to go so I put on my coat and went out the back door.

I didn't have a clue which way I was going. I was tired and petrified; it was like 11 pm. We tried hard not to be on the block really late at night. It was really scary because I was always afraid that the police would stop me and I would get arrested.

The way I was feeling, though, was that I would do anything to get just one more good score, including risking my freedom!

It was cold and extremely dark outside and I had such an uneasy feeling as I started walking up the block. I was actually so tired that I really couldn't walk fast. As I walked, I passed my mom's house.

I passed by my mom's house a lot when I was on the stroll because it sat one house from the corner of the main block. I really wanted to knock on the door because I was so tired and afraid, but I knew it would be pointless. Even if I heard someone come to the door, I would just hear them walk away again. I knew that sound all too well.

I had exhausted my attempts with my mom and she didn't let me in her house anymore. How could I blame her? The last time she let me in, I stole money from her purse. It's sad to admit, but if she let me in again during that time, I would probably have attempted to do it again. She did the right thing by keeping me out.

The sad truth is that I had alienated all my family and I especially missed my kids. My oldest two were grown and the baby girl was a teenager. I missed out on ten years of their life. I tried to maintain a relationship with them at the beginning of my addiction, but as it progressed, all bets were off. I couldn't face them and I believed they were better off without me.

My husband took my youngest daughter from me early in my addiction. She was lucky. My husband and I were separated at the time and I had taken her with me to live with my mom. I can still see her looking back at me from the backseat of the car as he drove away.

One of the most painful memories I recall happened on a sunny day. I saw my oldest daughter's car approaching while I was walking down the stroll looking for a trick. I had no time to hide, so I just turned my head in shame. I really hated myself for what I've done to my children. I really couldn't for the life of me understand how I could be so ruthless. I loved my kids, but sadly the drugs came first.

I left my son to fend for himself most of his pre-teen and teenage life. I showed up when I could, but for the most part, that was never. After high school, he was fed up and he moved to Florida. I totally lost track of him then. He is my only son and I let him down so much.

I wasn't always a bad mom: there was a time when my kids were my whole world and I would do anything for them. But once I met crack, everything changed.

My kids were not the only casualties: I even alienated my best friend I had known since third grade. The alienation came mostly from shame: I was a homeless drug addict and there was no time for meaningful relationships. Staying high helped me cope with their loss. So moving on, I needed a hit. After that walk down memory lane, I needed a hit bad; so bad that I was shaking!

TRICKED

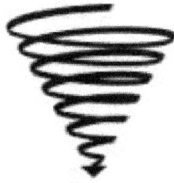

I continued to walk down the street towards the little store hoping to get some quick action. I saw a car pass me and hit the brakes, so I ran to catch up with it. I jumped in the front passenger seat.

When I got in I noticed there was a car seat in the back and it was a young guy driving with his window down smoking a cigarette. I had never seen him before, but I wasn't alarmed. I asked him what he was looking for and that it would be $100 upfront.

Strangely, he just continued to drive and didn't pay me. He seemed a little nervous, so I told him again $100. He continued driving and smoking his cigarette. We approached a street that I knew was a dead-end and I told him to make the turn. When we got to the end of the dead-end I told him again that it would be $100. He opened up his glove compartment. I thought he was getting the money out, but he pulled out a gun!

He instructed me to lay my seat all the way back. I was really shook but I had to think fast. He laid the gun on the center console and unzipped his pants. As he prepared to climb over on top of me, I told him to hold on while I get a condom out of my backpack. I remembered that I had recently purchased a lighter that looked like a small pistol when you pull the trigger the flame ignites. I pulled it out, thinking what did I have to lose? I never liked getting tricked so I had to try it! I pulled the pistol lighter out and put it straight to his temple.

Then, I quickly took his gun and threw it out of his open window. It worked; I was back in control! He was devastated as I held the pistol lighter to his temple. He began to apologize and cry, telling me that his wife had just had a baby and couldn't have sex. Blah, blah, blah. I was furious!

As I screamed, I instructed him to back all the way down to the dead-end of the street. Once we got to the street, I exited the car and screamed at him to never come on the block again. I told him if he did I would kill him. He sped off! I took a minute to collect myself. I was actually very proud of myself. I really couldn't believe that it worked.

I took a good look at the car and made a mental note of what he looked like so I could warn the other ladies and the dope boys about him. We always looked out for each other that way. Nevertheless, I was standing outside on the block in the same predicament—no crack and no money!

I really, really needed a hit. I cautiously continued my stroll. I wasn't really scared that he would come back, but I felt uneasy being on the main strip that late. It was around 1 am.

NOT MUCH ACTION

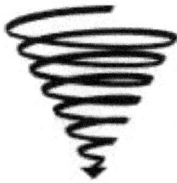

There were very few headlights on the road that early in the morning. I was on the main strip desperate! As the next set of headlights approached, I noticed that it was my friend driving his wife's van. I was relieved.

He pulled over to the curb and I quickly jumped in. He pulled off and headed to our normal spot, but when we got to the stoplight to make the turn, he gave me $7.00 and asked me to get out.

I pleaded with him to drop me off back at the house where I had left from the previous morning, but he wouldn't listen to me. He kept telling me to get out. I opened the door to get out and he told me to clean myself up and that he would look for me again later.

I was both embarrassed and devastated. He had put me out back on the main strip. It wasn't a good time to be on the main strip. I knew that the cops would be cruising at this time of the morning. I decided to give up on scoring again and just try to find somewhere to go inside.

From where he had put me out, I was only a block away from a friend's house. I had known him for years as well. He started out as just another customer that picked me up for some work, but as we got to know each other we became friends. He used to be an addict himself and he always told me that I didn't belong in the game.

I knew that if he was home, even if he didn't want to do anything, he might let me clean myself up and stay for a while. As I approached the house, I glanced down his long driveway and saw that his car was gone. My stomach sunk; my luck had run out! Now what was I supposed to do?

It had been such a good day, but I only had $7.00. I was tired, cold, hungry, and had nowhere to go.

I sat on his porch for a few minutes to collect my thoughts, but I knew I had to move on soon. While I was sitting on his porch I began to cry. I prayed and asked God to help me. I had the overwhelming feeling that I couldn't do this anymore; I was so tired of living like that. Then I got up and started walking back towards the main block. The quickest way to get anywhere was to get back on the main strip.

I thought that maybe if I made it back to Bird's house, he would let me in. At that point, I didn't care about the house's urine smell, I just wanted to be inside and to feel safe. Six blocks away from his house, I started walking in that direction.

RUN

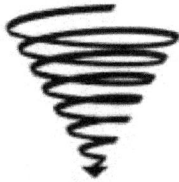

As I approached the little store, I saw a cop car parked in the parking lot and my heart started racing. I was courageous enough to walk past cops before and had no problem. I had even been stopped by the police while on the stroll before and given them some grand story that they believed and let me continue on the stroll. But this time was different. Very different!

The police car door opened and I heard the officer say my name—my maiden name. My heart dropped. I knew if I went to jail, I wouldn't get out. I had a *failure to appear* charge, a possession charge over my head, and I had drug paraphernalia on me. All I could think was RUN, so that's what I did!

Granted I had on four-inch heels which made running virtually impossible, but I ran as fast as I could. Nevertheless, I couldn't run far enough! I tripped and fell to the ground. As the officer stood over me, he warned me that back up was coming and if I tried to run again, they might not be as gracious and chase me. The outcome would be a lot different.

He helped me up and escorted me by the arm back to the police car. He asked me if I had anything on me and actually turned his head as I threw my stem away. He then handcuffed me and put me in the back of the police car.

This wasn't my first trip to jail, but I really wanted it to be my last. I was tired, so very tired. As I sat in the police car I actually prayed that I would never see the stroll again. The officer asked me how did I end up in my situation. I told him it all started as a "party", that turned out to be my worst nightmare. He sighed and I cried.

While in the back of the police car, all I could think about was the fact that I wouldn't be getting out anytime soon. I had previous charges, two felony possessions, and one failure to appear. With my track record, there was no way the judge would let me out on bail. I was hopeless and scared.

While in jail, I went from the local to the regional jail miles away, in a matter of weeks. At the regional jail, I had a cellmate whose story resembled my own. She had great aspirations of getting out and she spent every day researching drug programs that might accept inmates with drug charges. She was very excited when she found a specific program where she was certain we would be accepted. I pretended to be excited too but inside I was scared to death.

I was reluctant to leave jail. My past experiences had shown me that every time I got out of jail I went back to using. Quite frankly, I didn't want to risk it. In jail, I was safe—safe from myself!

When I got arrested on that early morning of December 1, 2006, that was my last day using and my first day of freedom from addiction. To most people, being locked up in jail wouldn't be considered freedom, but it was freedom for me. I was actually glad to be away from the streets of despair. I didn't have to try to find a place to sleep when I was tired and I could actually take a real bath. I didn't have to steal something to eat or wait for the local convenience store to throw out the day-old sandwiches and donuts.

Most of all, I didn't have to worry about walking up and down the street trying to get enough money to score. Yes, for me, jail was freedom and I was actually afraid to leave. I was afraid of going back to the stroll.

I had been locked up twice before and every time I got out, I went back to using. I couldn't stop! Every day in jail was better than being on the streets. No more turning tricks to get high. No more homelessness. No more self-degradation. No more humiliation! No more fear of the police! No more fear of getting in the wrong car and being raped or killed!

Jail was definitely freedom for me.

TRUE FREEDOM

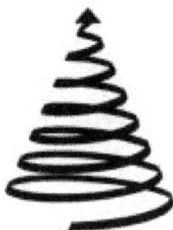

At my pre-trial hearing, I learned that I was facing a significant amount of time for felony drug possession and I could possibly be transferred out to a long-term facility. After court, I decided to start attending the weekly Bible Study meetings that the jail offered. At my third meeting, the Pastor was talking about hope and he referenced Jeremiah 29:11, NIV:

"For I know the plans I have for you, declares the Lord, plans to give you Hope and a future".

When I got back to my cell, I read that verse over and over. I began to believe that God had a plan for me.

After thinking about being transferred and considering how long I would be locked up, I decided to try the drug court program. I applied and was eventually interviewed by two intake officers. I was accepted.

After being in jail for three months, I was released into a drug court program in March of 2006. I had been in jail for three months and that was the longest I had been locked up. I was really happy to get out. Now if I could just stay clean.

To my surprise, this time being out of jail was different for me—my mom allowed me to move in with her. I went to the program and meetings every day. I found hope listening to people share their stories and, even though I was scared, I stayed clean one day at a time.

Living day to day without using was very difficult for me at first. I lived with my mom whose house was right off of the stroll. When I went outside, I would often see people I had used with. In between recovery meetings and the program, I stayed in the house where I was safe. Every day I watched the clock. I usually got home from the program around

4:00 and I couldn't wait until it was time to take my shower and go to bed.

Getting a job and starting a savings account was a program requirement. On the first application I filled out, I panicked when I got to the part about *check here if you have ever been convicted of a felony*. I couldn't check the box; I was overwhelmed with shame and despair. I balled the application up and threw it in the trash, but I knew this wouldn't work for me. After all, I had to get a job; it was a program requirement (get a job or go back to jail).

I continued to fill out applications and throw them away. Eventually, out of mere desperation, I checked the box and explained my felony. To my surprise, I got the job and I opened the required savings account.

When I received my first check, I broke out in a cold sweat and my hands began to shake. I was afraid. I was afraid of having cash in my possession. I was afraid of using again. I begin to cry. I stuffed the check in my purse and I went to a meeting and talked about how I was feeling. At the meeting, I found hope and gained the strength to go to the bank and make my deposit.

I deposited more than the required amount in my savings account and I took the rest home and gave it to my mom to hold for me. I wasn't ready to hold my own money or open a checking account and acquire a debit card. No, not yet!

Eventually, I overcame my fear of access to money and I was able to get a checking account and a debit card without the fear of using them. I remember when I placed the debit card in my wallet, I had such a sense of pride. When I think about it, it's kind of crazy because I was 47 years old and most people my age wouldn't have such pride over carrying a debit card, but for me, it was truly an accomplishment. It was one of the first obstacles that I had overcome and I was able to practice a learned principle of replacing my fear with faith.

MEDITATION

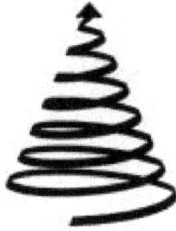

After two years, I completed the drug court program. Through counseling and meetings, I came to the realization that drugs were only a symptom of my problem. The core of my addiction was the need to alter my personal reality and my inability to live life on life's terms. Now came the true test—living clean without supervision.

I was so used to reporting in and random drug screens, I knew that I had to do what was right if I wanted to remain free. I wouldn't have that security on the outside; my life was totally in my hands.

I realized that even though I had been clean for two years, I had actually been living in survival mode.

Just doing what I had to do to get by, but I wasn't LIVING. I was afraid to get back out there and enjoy life. It was time for me to face my demons and ENJOY life. It was time for me to start living again.

I started attending church on a regular basis, building on my foundation of hope. It was important for me to replace my negative thoughts of self with the way that God saw me. The way God sees me has nothing to do with negativity, so I really had to meditate on that. It was easy for me to live in fear and worry about the future; that's was what I was used to. However, I found that meditation was the key to release me from worry. Meditation was the key to change my outlook on life.

The word meditate means to think about something over and over again. So I had to make a choice: either I could think about the things that worry me over and over again or I could think about positive things that were positive in my life over and over again. The choice was mine.

With some work, I began to dream a little. If I was going to spend every waking moment of the day thinking about something, why not use that time to think about the positive things like my future? I had to remember that God had promised me a future and hope, not doom and gloom. So I renewed my mind to the promises of God.

The best way that I found to renew my mind to the promises of God was through affirmations. I became my biggest cheerleader—I didn't wait for anyone to encourage me or affirm me. I began to affirm myself.

Affirmations became a very important part of my morning routine. With all that goes on in life, it's easy to hang your head and declare *What's the use*? Instead of hanging my head, I decided to keep my head up and declare what God said about me. Every morning to this day, I go into the bathroom, close the door and face the mirror, looking at myself, saying:

- At this moment, I choose to release the past and look forward to the good that awaits me.

- With each new breath, I inhale strength and exhale fear. I am learning that it is safe for me to heal and grow.

- At this moment, I choose to feel calm and peaceful. Everything is unfolding as it should.

- I will not fear because God is with me.

- ➢ Isaiah 41:10, NIV: So do not fear, for I am with you; do not be dismayed, for I am your God. I will strengthen you and help you; I will uphold you with my righteous right hand.

- I choose to fill my mind with positive, nurturing, and healing thoughts.

- There are no mistakes, only lessons to be learned, and I am doing the best I can.

- I will not faint at the sign of adversity:

  - ➢ Isaiah 40:31, KJV: But they that wait upon the Lord shall renew their strength; they shall mount up with wings as eagles; they shall run, and not be weary; and they shall walk, and not faint.

- God is always with me. I am strong and filled with courage.

  - ➢ Joshua 1:9, NIV: Have I not commanded you? Be strong and courageous. Do not be afraid; do not be discouraged, for the LORD your God will be with you wherever you go.

- I will not be anxious about anything.

  ➢ Philippians 5:6-7, NIV: Do not be anxious about anything, but in every situation, by prayer and petition, with thanksgiving, present your requests to God. And the peace of God, which transcends all understanding, will guard your hearts and your minds in Christ Jesus.

Affirmations give me a fresh start every day, a time to shake off every negative thing—doubt, self-loathing, hopelessness, and fear all have to go. Affirmations keep me positive in the midst of adversity. By the time I leave the mirror in the mornings, I have the strength of a Lion—I feel like I can do anything. Guess what? I CAN!

I am more than a conqueror. I know that I have a bright future and I am certain that God didn't bring me this far to leave me.

CONNECTIONS

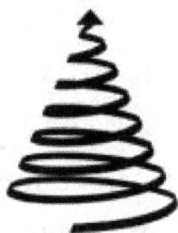

I love all people, but not all people have my best interest at heart. Toxic relationships breed toxic behavior and I had enough of toxic behavior when I was on the street. I am very careful about the company I keep. I can't hang around people with no goals and expect to achieve anything.

The people I allow in my circle are goal-oriented winners. I am blessed to still have my best friend from childhood in my life—we have been friends for over 50 years. I have a small circle of friends and I am careful with my words. I call my connections *favor connections* because I believe that the people that are in my life are there for my edification and support. This group of people has *favor* on their lives and I can see God in them. They are walking on one accord with God and are achieving things they could never achieve on their own. I am inspired by them to be a better person.

Being connected to people who have favor on their lives and are further along in their successes than I am, gives me the opportunity to learn and to grow. The favor that's on their lives actually flows down to me. I am able to see an increase in my blessings and success because of my positive connections.

It is very important to be connected to people that challenge you to be better instead of people who drain your energy and keep you stuck. I hang with the winners—people who are going places, people who want to take their lives to the next level, and people who have accomplished the dreams that I am pursuing.

One of the greatest connections that I have today is the connection with my family. The restoration of my family is an ongoing task—it definitely didn't happen overnight. I ran from my relationship with my husband for years after I got clean. I dated other people and even contemplated filing for divorce. However, I spoke to him one evening and asked him why he never divorced me. After hearing him reply, "Because I still love you", I was introduced to hope.

I could hear the pain of my past in my oldest daughter's voice when she spoke of seeing me walking down the street and watching me turning away from her. She told me that she often wished that I had died because she knew death would be far better than the life I was living.

There are other touching moments like visiting my son's home in Florida and having him come sit beside me and lay his head in my lap as we weep listening to Boyz to Men's song *Mama*. Or watching my youngest daughter still go to her dad for her needs and advice. Even though I'm back in her life now, my husband was a single parent to her for her most of her childhood.

I realize that my past mistakes were extremely devastating to my loved ones and I have been given the gift of forgiveness. Rebuilding these relationships is a daily blessing for me. I am challenged to stay present in their lives both physically and mentally. I am grateful for the opportunity to grow as a wife, mother, grandmother, and most recently, great-grandmother.

THERE IS HOPE

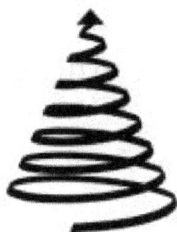

Jeremiah 29:11, NIV:

"For I know the plans I have for you, declares the Lord, plans to give you Hope and a future".

My journey has given me the greatest gift of my entire life—the Gift of Hope. I remember how hearing Jeremiah 29:11 completely changed my life when I was in jail. That scripture was the foundation for my true freedom. The word *hope* spoke volumes to me.

Hearing that scripture was the turning point for me. It was because of *hope* that I began to believe that I could have a better life. I really could have a better life! There is a possibility that this could work for me. Hope!

What does it mean to have hope? Listen, when I got locked up in December of 2006, I was at my lowest point—the pits of hopelessness. I truly believed there was no hope for me to live a life free from drug addiction. So to be given the gift of hope meant the world to me.

What hope meant to me was that:

- Maybe, just maybe, I had a chance.

- Maybe, just maybe, I could live a life free from drugs.

- Maybe, just maybe, I could have a future.

- Maybe, just maybe, I could live and not die.

I took hold of that *maybe*, that hope, and ran with it.

Today, I am *The Hope Dealer*, offering the same hope and future to others that were given to me. It is my desire to teach the masses, giving the gift of hope to those whose story resembles my own. Giving the gift of hope to those people that are otherwise on a downward spiral of hopelessness, gives my life purpose.

I desire to give the gift of hope to all people because we've all faced a demon that we surely thought would take us out. I can't promise anyone that they won't face any demons in this life, but I can certainly promise that there is **freedom**.

GOD'S GRACE

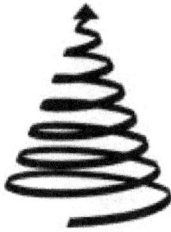

Growing up I was very inquisitive and I had many questions for my father concerning life. I was brought up in church—we were actually voted the church family of the year once. I was taught the difference between right and wrong and the preacher always talked about heaven and hell. I was very concerned about people going to heaven because I didn't want anyone to go to hell. My father was a Deacon at our church and a strong man of faith. I was very close to my dad.

As a child when I began to hear about or observe things in life that leaned toward the scale of being wrong, I would ask my dad so many questions.

- When someone commits murder can they go to heaven?

- What about that man on the news that robbed the bank can he go to heaven?

- Or the lady down at the store who was saying bad words, will she go to heaven?

And on and on. To all of these questions concerning right and wrong, my father would always give me the same response. He would look at me and say with a great big smile, "God's grace is sufficient." I can admit that as a child I didn't know what *grace* was, but I knew by my father's smile that it was a good thing.

God's grace is unearned, unmerited favor, a spiritual blessing of divine enablement. God's unmerited, unearned favor is adequate, or enough for us to receive every spiritual blessing that God has prepared for us. That means that I am not condemned for my past and I'm not condemned when I make a mistake even now. Nobody is perfect—we all need some unearned favor in our life, especially the kind that unlocks blessings of divine enablement. Blessings of divine enablement are blessings to succeed at everything you do! So that's why my dad answered me saying, "God's grace is sufficient." He knew that the grace of God was adequate to save those who missed the mark and bless them with a future.

Jeremiah 1:5 is one of my favorite meditational scriptures—it reminds me that before God even formed me in the womb of my mother, He knew and approved of me. He knew that I would be his chosen instrument before I was even born and he separated me and set me apart, dedicating and appointing me to be His spokesperson to the nations. He did all of this before I was even born. My mistakes were no surprise to Him because He knew the master plan would be for His glory and His grace was sufficient to bring me out of every storm.

My life journey thus far has shown me that God's grace is truly sufficient. I know that it is only because of God's grace that I survived the streets and the deepest, darkest parts of my addiction. I know that it is only because of God's grace that I have been given a future and hope wherein I can help others. The same grace that was extended to me is available to everyone and I am a willing vessel to carry that message. The message of freedom, the message of hope, the message of a future for those who otherwise feel hopeless and unworthy.

It amazes me that when God laid out the plan for my life, He didn't just give me enough to get by, but He supplied me with an abundance of tools for success. I have learned not to get comfortable where I am, but to continue to strive for more. This *more* is not necessarily for my own selfish needs, but the needs of others.

I know that God supplies my needs in abundance because He wants me to help someone else to see Him the way that I see Him. Today I take the limits off of my dreams and I dare to dream big because I know I serve a big God. He is the God of more than enough and I plan to tap into all that He has for me. In this way, I can lead others to know Him and to also live in abundance. God is propelling me into my purpose and to that I say, "Full steam ahead. No turning back!"

STAY FOCUSED

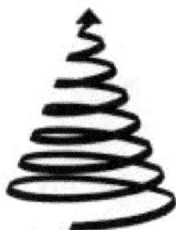

I'm so excited about where this journey is taking me and, the good news is, this is only the beginning. The most important thing is to stay focused on who God has called me to be. My journey is not anyone else's journey, it is strictly my own.

My past has made my vision clear and I am focused on using every part of my journey to help someone else and, in turn, brighten my future. Staying focused is not as easy as it sounds—it requires work and perseverance.

When I first got clean, I was lost. I had no idea who I was and what my purpose was in life. I spent all of my time trying to be what other people said I should be. If I aspired to apply for one job and someone said I would be better at something else, I went with what they said. I like to wear my hair long, but if someone said I would look better with short hair, I'd wear it short. I love makeup, but if someone told me not to wear makeup, I didn't wear makeup, and so on. I was miserable and frustrated trying to please other people and ultimately lost myself.

It was only after I started meditating and becoming comfortable with myself that I was able to be myself and go after the goals and desires that God had placed on my heart. I realize today that there's an anointing on my life and that anointing is to be who God has called me to be. In doing so, I find myself happy and fulfilled, not frustrated, and empty. I am more confident every day and I see the favor of God working for me.

Being who you are requires boldness. I use to be easily influenced because I wanted other people to accept me even with the blaring mistakes that I had made. I felt as if I had to accept less because I wasn't worthy of more and people constantly brought up my past. However today I see things differently, when I am reminded of my past mistakes and baited into believing that I will never be anything, I fight back. I use my affirmations and I declare that I am who God my creator says I am. I am the apple of his eye, created in His image. I am in right standing with him, so the opinions of others don't matter. When God is for me no one can stand against me.

I accept myself for who I am, and I know that I am worthy of good things in life. With this attitude, I am able to stay focused and move forward and fulfill my purpose on this earth. I know that there will be obstacles along the way, but I believe that long as I stay focused and keep the right attitude I will be able to overcome them all.

FULFILLING MY PURPOSE

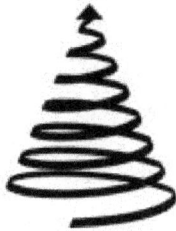

One of the biggest decisions that I made after getting clean was to go back to college. I went to college right after high school but I didn't finish. Instead, I got pregnant and left school in my third year. So finishing school had been something that I had put on the back burner, but I always thought that one day I would be able to go back.

I remember the day I decided to go back to school. My oldest daughter came to my room and told me that I am a great counselor. She said I had given her hope in what seemed to be hopeless situations. She went on to tell me that I had a gift that should be shared with the world. It was an affirmation for me because God had been dealing with me about speaking to the nation, sharing my story so that others might have hope in what otherwise seems to be a hopeless world. So I decided that it was time to go back to school and focus on religious studies, evangelism. Evangelism means being a witness for God and that was certainly right up my alley.

Yes, I was afraid, but I decided to do it afraid. I decided not to let my fear keep me from my destiny. I decided to do it afraid and I received my Bachelor of Science Degree in Religious Studies on December 14, 2018. I finished with honors, Magna Cum Laude. I never would have thought that I had enough brain cells left after what I put my body through to be able to think straight enough to even finish college, let alone with honors, but God.

I must admit that even after having success in college, the chains of unworthiness still had me bound. After finishing, I immediately began to ask myself why I wasted my time. Thank God for His word.

Because of the word of God, I was able to break the chains of unworthiness and move on. I realized that we all have forces trying to hold us back—chains that try to restrict us from moving forward to our destinations. For me, it was chains of unworthiness and guilt.

I had a bad habit of beating myself up for my past mistakes, but the good news is that God is a chain breaker. I could hear him saying to me, "This is your time to be free and it is your destiny to go through life without anything limiting you. It is your destiny to be free. I came to give your life and not just an ordinary life – an abundant life".

I realize today that I never really needed a professional certification to do what God has called me to do. My degree is merely an added bonus because I didn't have to wait for anyone to certify, approve, or validate me. All I needed to do was use the gift that my life journey had given me, my testimony. That is why when I look back over my life and if I had it to do all over again, I can sincerely say I wouldn't change a thing. If it had not been for the dark places on my journey, I wouldn't have my life-saving testimony. A testimony of God's grace and mercy.

Fulfilling God's purpose for my life is the most important thing that I can do to show my gratitude for all that He has done for me. As a servant of the Most

High, I have been called to share the word of God with both the saved and the lost. The clear message about a future and hope, not death but eternal life.

I have been given the gift to defeat demons and cast down strongholds in the name of Jesus. I have accepted my calling without fear because I know that He who called me makes no mistakes and I stand as a living witness of his undying mercy. I was ordained as a Minister of the Gospel on November 3, 2019. Fittingly, I have been assigned to the addiction ministry at my church and I am eager to start.

Unfortunately, in March of 2020, everyone's life changed. There was an outbreak of a pandemic called the coronavirus, also known as COVID-19. There have been insurmountable deaths and a worldwide quarantine causing churches, businesses, and schools to close, some permanently. A lot of people lost jobs and no one can go out in public without wearing a mask. My church is now doing ministry via Facebook and YouTube. I serve as an "e-minister" and the launch of the Addiction Ministry has been postponed.

I look forward to the end of the COVID-19 pandemic so I can implement the addiction ministry in full force. With the increased amount of relapse that has happened as a direct result of the pandemic, this ministry is needed now more than ever. In preparation for the near future, I am diligently working with my best friend to start a podcast to address many issues facing our society including addiction and family caregivers.

MOVING FORWARD

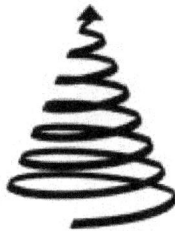

One of the hardest realizations that I have had on this journey is that not everyone is going to be my biggest cheerleader. I would love to tell you that all of my family and acquaintances are celebrating with me as I move forward in my life purpose, but that is not the case. For some reason, some just can't handle my success or they don't understand how I could be successful after the past mistakes that I have made. Moreover, they may wonder how God could bless me so abundantly when I had such an awful past and they have lived a "model" life and they are struggling. However, to that I say, you don't know my God. God is no respecter of person—His blessings are available to us all.

Nevertheless, I am well aware of my critics, those who try to smother my dreams, but they will not stop me. Unless they are offering constructive criticism for my edification and growth, critics don't matter to me. I have learned that in order for criticism to be constructive it must meet four requirements:

1. It should be given in a way that indicates that the person cares about your well-being and success

2. It should come from someone you respect and look up to

3. It should be on target offering specific guidance for your personal growth and improvement

4. It should be a match for your own emotions and motivation.

Otherwise, people's opinions of you are none of your business. I realize that my destiny is too great to be distracted by people who may never affirm me. Critics only motivate me to be my best self—it's God's opinion of me and my opinion of myself that really matters. Today I love me—I think that I am pretty awesome and it is my desire to grow not to shrink. No matter what, I must never lose sight of the purpose that God has planted on the inside of me.

I strive to move forward to greatness even in the midst of criticism. To be great even in the midst of criticism requires me to exercise the art of forgiveness. I have learned to not hold grudges but pray for my critics. I pray that they find peace and success in every area of their lives. As I stay focused on doing what is right, God is able to honor and promote me to go higher and higher. I recognize that my promotion comes from God, not from man.

After getting clean in 2006, I have been blessed to work as a camera technician, beauty advisor, fashion model, assistant store manager, and even store manager. However, caring for my mom is the best, most fulfilling, and challenging thing that I have been blessed to do thus far.

My mom lives with me and my husband now—she was diagnosed with dementia and I was ultimately granted guardianship and conservatorship for her.

When we moved mom in, I initially installed a camera and hired caregivers to come into my home and take care of her while I worked. However, after watching the caregiver sit on her phone most of the day, and then having another caregiver show up with alcohol on her breath, I quickly decided to give my two-weeks' notice and take care of my mom myself.

I learned a lot from my mom's nurses and caregivers at rehab before she came to live with us, so I was confident in becoming my mom's full-time caregiver. In addition, I decided to enroll in caregiver classes and I received my caregiver certificate and license. After spending the past ten years in retail management, I am now a licensed full-time caregiver.

Every morning when I get up, I hurry into the kitchen to put some applesauce in the pills my husband crushed up the night before for mom's morning meds. I grab her bottled water and a high-calorie breakfast drink before going into her room. When I open her door, I see mom squeeze her eyes close tightly as she pretends that she is still asleep, her way of saying *don't bother me*. Nevertheless, I enter and tell her *good morning*. Sometimes she responds and sometimes she doesn't. If it's a good day, mom responds with a *good morning* and we proceed with our daily routine.

A lot has changed over the past fourteen years. I never thought that I would be living a life free from active addiction or taking care of my mom. When I was using, I always thought that I would die that way. I had tried to stop using numerous times during my ten years of active addiction, but I would pick back up again after a short period of time. It was a vicious cycle of hopelessness. I learned to adapt to that way of life and I thought I might as well make the best of it and be the best at the game. Somehow, in my crazy thinking, I made myself believe that as long as I was able to keep getting high and find somewhere to go, I would be alright.

The truth was, I would never be alright—I grew more hopeless every day of my ten-year downward spiral on the street. Through my journey, I was beaten, kidnapped, thrown out of a car, held at gunpoint, raped, and more. I had no idea how I survived; it was definitely God's protection.

When I was in the midst of addiction, I almost stopped believing in God because I would always question how He could let me go through all of that. What I realize today is that it was God's grace that kept me. It was only because of His undying mercy that I am here to tell my story today. My journey to freedom has taught me that as long as you have breath, there is always hope. There is no such thing as a hopeless situation.

No, I wouldn't change anything about my story. It may seem crazy but I know that my journey made me the person that I am today. I believe that I have been pushed into my purpose by my pain—a purpose that is bigger than anything I had ever imagined.

I am a strong resilient woman, full of hope and vigor. A passionate loving woman, full of grace and hope. I am a grateful person with compassion for those who have not found freedom. No longer am I girded by hopelessness and despair. I have a purpose! I have a posture of gratitude. It is because of my gratitude that I was compelled to share my journey.

Many people looking at me today would never believe where God has brought me from, yet this narrative thus far has been only a glimpse at my journey and I certainly do not want to return to my dark place. If anyone had told me fourteen years ago when I began this journey that I would have the love and respect of my family and friends again; that I would be reunited with my husband of 37 years; that I would be in contact with my children on a regular basis; and that I would be an ordained minister, I would have surely thought they had lost their entire mind. However, God had a plan all along.

Ultimately, my journey has brought me to a place where I can help countless people by sharing my story. I am grateful because I realize that many people who have gone through the same situation that I went through didn't make it, but I did and I won't let the sparing of my life be in vain. Today my purpose in life is being fulfilled and taking steps to be a positive difference in the lives of others. On this downward spiral to freedom, I've gone from being totally selfish to being selfless. I recognize the needs of other people before my own today and that's a real switch up. That's actually real freedom for me, freedom from self.

KEEP YOUR GUARD UP

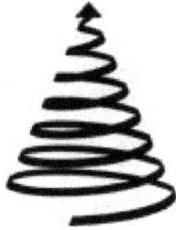

There are plenty of opportunities in life to get upset or walk around frustrated, but I choose to remain secure in my joy because pouting gets me nowhere. I truly believe that I control my own joy—it was given to me by God, therefore, no one can take it from me. However, I can give it away so I have to be very mindful of situations that would cause me to feel down in the dumps. Some of these situations are unavoidable, however, the way that I react to them is totally up to me. I have a choice and I choose happiness. I choose to keep my joy! One of my favorite sayings is "No joy snatching allowed."

Ultimately, life is way too short to live frustrated, upset about things that you and others have no control over. I have learned to let people have their opinions because they are entitled to them, but I also have the right to ignore them. People even have the right to be rude, but the important thing for me to remember is that I have the right to stay happy. I am entitled to peace and joy.

Proverbs 4:23, NIV is my no joy snatching reminder, it says:

> "Above all else, guard your heart, for everything you do flows from it..."

I refuse to let insignificant things like other people's moods, someone talking about me, my children or grandchildren getting on my nerves, my husband's snoring, or anything steal my joy. I make a decision every morning to be joyful and, when I'm tempted to get upset, I remind myself that I have the power. I have the power to keep my joy or to give it away.

I have learned to walk in freedom and not be discouraged by this process called living life on my terms. It's all a preparation process—every struggle that I go through, every disappointment, and every delay is making me stronger. As long as I keep the right attitude, every situation I encounter can be used to build my character and make me a better person. I am grateful for both the thorns and roses—I see the beauty in both. Losing my joy is one of the easiest ways to give up on moving forward. So I choose to stay in the process; I choose to keep moving forward.

One of the greatest opportunities that I have had on this journey has been to enjoy the small things in life. I have learned not to miss the wonderful blessings of the present season in my life by wishing I had more or complaining. The real joy in my life comes from the simple things:

- watching my grandchildren grow up

- taking walks with my husband

- watching television with my mom

- talking on the phone with my son

- watching my daughters' dance

- laughing at my son's jokes

- staring up at the stars at night

I don't have to have big vacations or lots of money to enjoy life. I use to believe that happiness was in material things. Don't get me wrong, there is nothing wrong with a new car or a beautiful new diamond ring, but learning how to enjoy the simple things in life has given me a new perspective on happiness.

True happiness is seeing the good in others and helping them see the good in themselves. True happiness is knowing that God has me in the palm of his hand and my future is bright. True happiness is the freedom to live and falling more in love with life every day. True happiness is gratitude for where I've been and renewed hope for where I'm going. True happiness is never giving up, realizing the best is yet to come!

THE JOURNEY CONTINUES

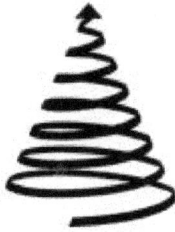

I know that my life is more fulfilling because of my relationship with God. It would be so easy to take care of my physical and emotional well-being and overlook my spiritual side. However, I believe that it was God that breathed this life into me, and ultimately He holds the key to my purpose and my future. Therefore, the most important part of my being is the spiritual side. When I put God first, His favor will take me where I could not possibly go on my own.

When I get up in the morning, God is the first thing on my mind and I thank Him for another day. I make sure that I prioritize God over everything else in my life because I know without Him nothing else would be possible. I make a point of meditating on His word daily. I meditate on His promises and what He wants for my life. This keeps my mind filled with hope on a daily basis. I know that by doing this I will have successful outcomes in every area of my life.

As I sit here watching television with my mom, I am grateful. My life is nothing short of a miracle—God has given me more than I could ever imagine. I remember believing that I would die in active addiction and now my life has meaning. I know that God will provide me with a long life. I truly pray that my life story will give hope to others. I know that my father is looking down on me and He is pleased with the person that I have become.

I am living proof that God doesn't want to just rescue you from your mess, He wants to give you another chance to get to where you're supposed to be. The mistakes that I made did not disqualify me from having a bright future. God is the God of a second chance and He has given me the opportunity to fulfill His best plan for my life.

The good news is that no matter the challenges that come up in my life, I don't end up defeated in failure and disappointment. I will always end in victory, fulfilling my destiny. Even in the midst of a very insecure world, I can rest in the security of knowing that my end has been set, knowing that God will always cause me to triumph.

Today, I can live in peace knowing that in the end, all things are going to work to my advantage. God already has an expected end for me. As long as I keep moving forward, He'll work it all together for my good and His glory. Ultimately, God has already established my victory and I will never give up!

LIVING MY BEST LIFE

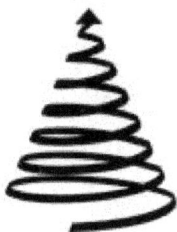

Recognizing that I have been set apart for God's glory has been truly freeing and motivating for me. What does it mean to be set apart? Deuteronomy 14:2 tells me that I have been set apart as holy to the LORD your God and He has chosen me from all the nations of the earth to be His own special treasure.

One of the biggest things that I had to overcome after being free from active addiction was the pressure to fit in—the need to do what everybody else was doing. By developing a personal relationship with God, I have discovered that I am not like anyone else, I am unique. God created me for a purpose that is uniquely my own. I have been set apart for his glory.

I don't find it necessary to compromise anymore. I remember when I first got clean, people would try to make me feel weak or less than because I didn't do the things that they did. I didn't want to go out and party. I didn't want to talk about other people or play the people-pleasing games. I often felt like an outcast and alone. Today I realize that it took a lot of courage for me to be myself. It took a lot of courage to be different and not to compromise. I'm actually not weak at all—I'm very strong and I won't be deceived into thinking otherwise. It's okay to be different, it's okay to be me.

Throughout life, it is very important to hold on to hope and not compromise because the truth of the matter is there will always be forces that will try to hold you back. I call them the chains of restriction. The chains of guilt have been my biggest enemy. I am always reminded of my past mistakes. I have also dealt with the chains of depression—dark clouds that follow me around, causing me to lose focus.

Low self-esteem is another chain that has often told me that I would never be anything and I would never accomplish anything. But there is good news: God is a chain breaker and He is saying,

"This is your time to be free. It is not your destiny to go through life with something limiting you."

When I let that take root in my spirit, every chain that was holding me back was BROKEN.

The things that held me back for years no longer have power over me. That's what happens when God shows up—He gives you a new way to live. I am so grateful because I have been given freedom and hope. It's a new day for me, a day of security and wholeness. No longer do I have to live in fear of myself and allow my insecurity and low self-esteem to run my life. I am totally free from those chains!

Addiction no longer has a hold over me because I recognize the root cause of my addiction was me and a new me has been born. I am well equipped to weather any storm. That's what happens when you put your complete trust in God, the chain breaker sets you free.

One of the greatest things that I have learned about God is that He is all-knowing. God already knows about everything I will go through in life— every hurt, every loss, and every mistake that I will make, God knows about it all. In His infinite wisdom, for every setback, He has arranged a comeback. I have been given a new beginning for every failure and restoration for everything I lost.

God has given me beauty for ashes. My journey has not been easy, but through my downward spiral, I have found freedom! I am living my best life.

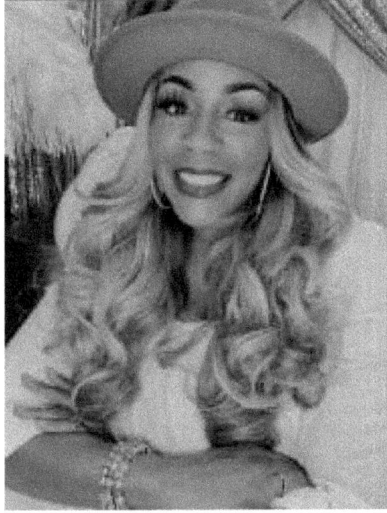

ABOUT THE AUTHOR

Growing up, Maria Roberts had many dreams and aspirations. As a child, she dreamed of being a princess, living in a big castle. As a young adult, she aspired to become a supermodel and travel the world. She attended college with the ambition of working in the juvenile justice field.

Never in her wildest dreams did she imagine the journey that life would take her on. Being the middle child of a school teacher and small business owner, Maria never yearned to be a drug addict.

My Downward Spiral to Freedom gives an up close look at a believer's journey from active addiction to freedom; from once desiring death to ultimately finding hope.